# STRENGTH TRAINING FOR SENIORS

# An Easy & Complete Step By Step Guide For YOU

# Table of Contents

**CHAPTER ONE: Why Strength Training?** ............................................. 5

    What the Medical Community Says About Strength Training for Seniors ................................................................................................ 7

    Relief from Arthritis ............................................................................ 8

    Improved Balance .............................................................................. 8

    Stronger Bones .................................................................................. 9

    Stronger Backs and Lungs ................................................................ 10

    Weight and Glucose Control ............................................................ 10

    Improved Emotional Makeup and Sleep .......................................... 11

    Stronger Heart ................................................................................. 12

    Warding off Dementia ..................................................................... 13

    Improved Ability to Perform Daily Tasks ......................................... 14

    More Likely to Continue Living Independently ............................... 15

    Testimonials .................................................................................... 16

    David Ratherdale, 65, with Type II Diabetes ................................... 17

    Harold Moss, 67, Cancer Survivor ................................................... 17

    T. Boone Pickens, 83, Billionaire Investor ....................................... 18

**CHAPTER TWO: A Program for Strength Training** ............................ 20

    How Much Time Per Week Will Strength Training Require? .......... 21

| | |
|---|---|
| What Counts as Strength Training and Aerobic Activity? | 22 |
| What You Will Need | 23 |
| Helpful Steps before You Start Moving | 24 |
| **CHAPTER THREE: SUGGESTED EXERCISES AND APPROACH** | **28** |
| Starter Exercises | 29 |
| Exercises for Those Ready to Use Weights | 31 |
| Additional Exercises | 34 |
| Stretching Exercises | 41 |
| **CHAPTER FOUR: MAKING PROGRESS** | **44** |
| Final Words | 46 |
| **SOURCES** | **48** |

# CHAPTER ONE

## Why Strength Training?

"Strength training" and "seniors" does not sound like a probable match, but in fact it is a match made in heaven. The mere thought of people who are past their physical prime pumping iron might seem vain or ludicrous, but millions of seniors are discovering the manifold benefits of strength training, and the medical community continues to produce studies showing that those who dare to incorporate strength training in their weekly routines gain all sorts of physical and emotional benefits.

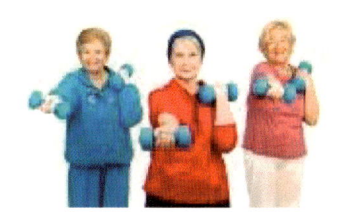

Unfortunately, many seniors discover the wonders of strength training while doing rehabilitation after a surgery or a fall. You don't have to wait until you experience a health crisis to begin doing strength training. In fact, starting a regular strength training program could prevent many of the crises that force seniors to do workouts with weights.

As more and more people live to older ages, more and more practices formerly thought of as being just for young people are creeping into older age categories as well. Seniors sky dive, seniors ski, seniors dance and seniors even get married and go on honeymoons. There's no reason why you as a senior cannot take up a strength training regimen, and it might not take as long as you think.

As more seniors begin to do strength training, they are finding that they feel better, look better and, in many cases, they are living longer as they get stronger and fitter. If the thought of any kind of exercise makes you feel a little ill, take heart. You can design your own program with the types of exercises that you enjoy and tone the parts of your body that you care about most.

Forget the images you have of muscle-bound men in Speedo swimsuits prancing around a gym or on stage during a body-building contest. Think instead of a group of happy seniors lifting light weights at a community center or in a hospital rehab room. Strength training is for all ages once the bones can sustain the strain (usually in pre-teen years), and its benefits accrue no matter how old you are (or feel).

Sure, there are some seniors that scoff at all forms of exercise. They recommend a diet of cigarettes and strong Scotch to grow old, but the ones who have followed such regimens for years and passed away before their time are not around to critique the merits of strength training. It's probably best to heed the wisdom of the medical community when considering whether or not you will begin a strength training program.

We thus turn to the studies that have been done touting the benefits of strength training for seniors. In the pages that follow, you should be able to find all of the motivation needed to get off the couch and grasp a dumbbell or two.

## What the Medical Community Says About Strength Training for Seniors

Several research studies have been done in the past decade, and they all proclaim the benefits of strength training for seniors. One of the key findings of these studies is that strength training can be quite beneficial even for those seniors who are not in ideal health. In other words, you don't have to look like Jack LaLane in his prime to do strength training. You can even be wheelchair-bound and still gain significant benefits from strength training. In fact, people with particular physical challenges, such as heart disease or arthritis, can gain the most from lifting weights a few times per week.[1]

And, of course, all of these wonderful byproducts of strength training are not limited to men—women should also follow a program of strength training combined with regular aerobic exercise. Furthermore, the gains that people make from strength training are not limited to the physical realm; seniors that engage in such exercise report outstanding progress in their mental and emotional health as well.[2]

For starters, let's consider the many medical conditions that can have their signs and symptoms reduced by consistent strength training:

- Arthritis
- Poor balance
- Diabetes
- Osteoporosis
- Obesity
- Back pain
- Breathing problems
- Depression

---

[1] Retrieved 12/29/12 from http://www.cdc.gov/physicalactivity/growingstronger/why/index.html
[2] Ibid

- Dementia

That's a list that strikes a chord with most seniors, in at least one area or more. How exactly does strength training help in these areas? Here are the details:

### Relief from Arthritis

A recent Tufts University study showed that strength training decreased pain from knee osteoarthritis by 43% as a result of a 16-week workout program for senior men and women. The subjects also reported increased muscle strength and physical performance while reducing the signs and symptoms of arthritis.

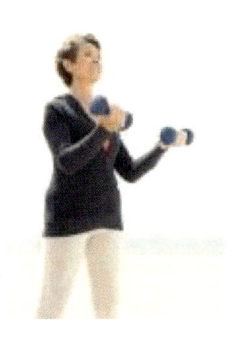

The most significant conclusion of the study? Strength training was at least as effective as medications in reducing the pain of arthritis.[3] The old adage "no pain, no gain" has to be modified in this instance. When it comes to seniors and strength training, the motto should be "lift a little, lose the pain," which seems a bit counterintuitive but has nonetheless been proven true in several studies.

### Improved Balance

Any senior can tell you that one of the most frustrating changes that occur when someone grows old is a loss of balance and flexibility, which often result in falls, broken bones and all sorts of other

---

[3] Ibid

complications, even death. How many of us have had an older relative fall and break a bone? Just about everyone! Unfortunately, some seniors are never the same after such a fall.

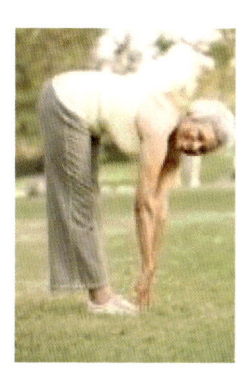

Strength training can help in this area as well. A study in New Zealand found that women aged 80 and older saw a 40% drop in the number of falls they had as a result of strength and balance training.[4] Strength training doesn't just build big biceps and other muscles. It increases flexibility, which helps balance, which means fewer falls and healthier golden years.

## Stronger Bones

Strength training also does more than impact the muscles involved. It actually can increase bone density, thus lowering the incidence of fracture—great news for seniors that often suffer from brittle bones and do tumble more than the general population.

Another Tufts University study conducted in 1994 showed that strength training significantly increased bone density in women aged 50-70.[5]

---

[4] Ibid
[5] Ibid

## Stronger Backs and Lungs

Specific strength training exercises can target the abdomen and chest muscles, resulting in more normal breathing patterns for longer periods of time, which means a lower incidence of chronic obstructive pulmonary disease.

In addition, the lower back, a common trouble spot for seniors, can be strengthened and made less painful through specific strength training movements that focus on the lumbar and sacral area.[6]

## Weight and Glucose Control

Obesity gains ground by the day in the United States and other countries. It has particularly harmful consequences for seniors, whose bodies are less able to handle extra weight and whose more vulnerable emotions can be particularly damaged by the self-image issues that result from a grossly overweight body.

Any trainer can tell you that strength training can help in this area because muscle consumes calories and does a better job of that as they are taxed and stretched. On average, a person's metabolism takes a 15% jump when that person practices consistent strength training.[7]

In addition, strength training can give renewed hope to those who battle diabetes. It not only helps with weight control, it can also do battle with glucose levels. That's more good news for the millions of Americans that have type II diabetes, a number that has mushroomed by 300% in the past 40 years.[8]

---

[6] Retrieved 12/29/12 from http://www.eldergym.com/elderly-strength.html
[7] Retrieved 12/29/12 from http://www.cdc.gov/physicalactivity/growingstronger/why/index.html
[8] Ibid

People with diabetes face an entire host of complications from the condition, including heart and renal disease, as well as blindness. Diabetes is, in fact, the leading cause of blindness in older adults. Strength training can not only build muscle and bone strength, it can perhaps have the additional indirect benefit of controlling diabetes and thus keeping your eyes functioning as they should, deep into your senior years.

A recent study of Hispanic men and women revealed that 16 weeks of strength training helped them to control their glucose levels about as well as medication. The participants also shed body fat and felt happier and more self-confident.[9] It makes you wonder why anyone would be opposed to strength training, given the sheaves of medical evidence that trumpet its multitude of benefits.

## Improved Emotional Makeup and Sleep

Anyone who has lived on planet Earth knows that our minds and bodies are intimately linked. When our bodies feel good and healthy, we are much more likely to be content or happy. Conversely, when we are sick or tired, our emotions often take a nosedive as well.

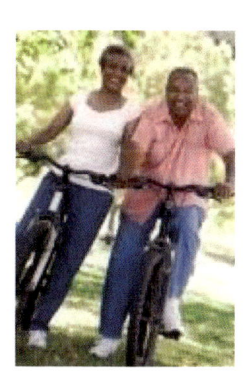

---

[9] Ibid

Sleep also figures into this equation, doesn't it? When we are not sleeping well we drag through each day until we reach a point of exhaustion and find ourselves constantly angry and feeling negative.

Strength training can help to maintain this optimal balance between mind and body and ensure that restful sleep is a regular part of our lives, not an elusive condition meant for others.

Strength training among people of all ages builds self-esteem and the likelihood of falling asleep soon after the head hits the pillow. Researchers are still working on the connection between strength training and the mind, trying to figure out why it is as effective as medication in relieving depression. It is probably a combination of improved self-image and chemical changes in the brain.[10]

After you admire yourself in the mirror and turn in for the night after another session of strength training, you will almost certainly sleep deeply for a longer period of time. Again, strength training assists sleep as well as medication, for a fraction of the cost.

**Stronger Heart**

There's a reason why the American Heart Association has recommended strength training as a prime way to reduce the risk of heart disease—because it works. Cardiac patients gain not only strength and flexibility, they improve their aerobic capacity when doing strength training three times per week. A leaner body enables your heart to work more efficiently, thus improving its chance of working well for a longer period of time. For these reasons, strength training is included as an integral part of cardiac rehabilitation programs in far more cases than even a couple of decades ago.

---

[10] Ibid

## Warding off Dementia

If you were to ever poll a group of seniors, or even those just ascending into middle age, about their greatest fear, dementia would certainly capture one of the top spots. Recent studies have shown that strength training can even help to ward off this great enemy of seniors.

Teresa Liu-Ambrose, assistant professor in the Department of Physical Therapy at the University of British Columbia, co-authored a study on the connection between weight lifting and slower loss of memory. One of the surprising findings of the study was that strength training did even more for staving off memory loss than aerobics-based activity.[11]

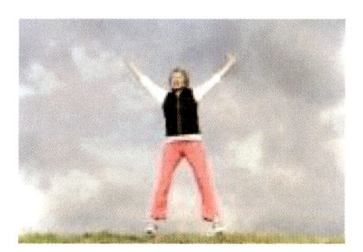

"Most studies have looked at aerobics training, but this study compares both aerobic and strength training," Liu-Ambrose said. "And among people who don't yet have dementia but are already at a high risk in terms of mild memory and executive function impairment, our study shows that strength training, but not aerobics training, does have benefits for cognition," she added.[12]

The study focused on women between 70 and 80 years old who were deemed to have probable mild cognitive impairment. The women did

---

[11] "Strength Training May Give Boost to Seniors' Brains," by Alan Mozes, retrieved 12/29/12 from http://health.usnews.com/health-news/news/articles/2012/04/23/strength-training-may-give-boost-to-seniors-brains
[12] Ibid

strength training for one hour, two days per week, over a six-month period. The women who did strength training outperformed others in the study that did walking or balance and toning classes, achieving "significant" cognitive improvement.[13]

That improvement resulted from activity changes that were noted in three parts of the brain's cortex, changes not seen in the other two groups that exercised. The study's authors were hesitant to promise the same differences among men or younger women.

As for why lifting weights did more for the brain than walking or balance exercises, Liu-Ambrose could only guess: "It could be that resistance training requires more learning and monitoring by its very nature," she said. "If you're lifting weights you have to monitor your sets, your reps, you use weight machines and you have to adjust the seat, etc. ...But at this point we don't have a clear idea of what's going on at the mechanistic level."[14]

**Improved Ability to Perform Daily Tasks**

Beyond the good work battling disease and debilitating conditions that strength training does for its practitioners, it also logically improves even the menial daily life of the average senior. In other words, you don't have to have a heart condition or diabetes to benefit immeasurably from regular strength training.

The esteemed Cochrane Collaboration, an international non-profit organization that focuses on health, has compiled a great deal of evidence proving that strength training helps seniors to walk, climb

---

[13] Ibid
[14] Ibid

steps and even get out of a chair far more easily than for those who do not practice strength training.[15]

Dr. Chiung-ju Liu of the Department of Occupational Therapy at Indiana University-Purdue University Indianapolis, looked at 121 trials involving 6,700 participants between the ages of 60 and 80 and found that adults that exercised two or three times per week consistently outperformed those who didn't as both groups did common daily movements, such as getting out of a chair, etc. The ones who did strength training also reported lower levels of pain from osteoarthritis.

The chief surprise of the study was that even people aged 80 can experience significant gains in ease of motion and strength through training.[16]

## More Likely to Continue Living Independently

Part of the obvious benefit of being able to perform routine tasks more easily and ward off dementia is the prospect of living independently for as long as possible. A year-long study in Canada has established a link between strength training and independent living, the goal of almost any senior that you talk to.[17]

---

[15] "Seniors Benefit from Strength Training" by Kurt Ullman, retrieved 12/29/12 from http://www.cfah.org/hbns/archives/getDocument.cfm?documentID=2091.
[16] Ibid
[17] "Strength Training for Seniors Provides Sustained Cognitive Function and Economic Benefits," retrieved from http://www.publicaffairs.ubc.ca/2010/12/13/strength-training-for-seniors-provides-sustained-cognitive-function-and-economic-benefits-vancouver-coastal-health-ubc-research/

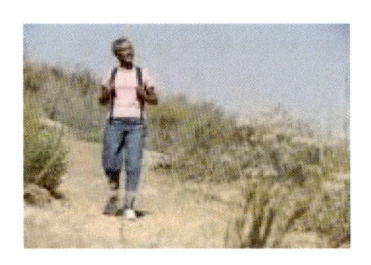

The study found that seniors who did strength training during the year of study showed "sustained cognitive benefits." The study was noteworthy in that it proved the savings to Canada's national healthcare system, as it built on earlier studies that had already established a link between once- or twice-weekly strength training exercises and improved executive cognitive function in women between 65 and 75. Such executive functions are absolutely necessary to living independently.[18]

In addition, the study showed that the economic benefits from strength training continued a full year after the program's end, as participants needed less health care and fell far less frequently. The study also hinted (curiously) that once-a-week strength training might be the correct amount for seniors in the upper echelon of age.[19]

## Testimonials

So, what does strength training for a senior look like in the real world? Does it include only those who were elite athletes and love to exercise, or can it encompass those who even hate to sweat and have never been very athletic?

Here are a couple of testimonials from seniors who have shared their story with the Centers for Disease Control and Prevention.[20] They

---

[18] Ibid

[19] Ibid

[20] Retrieved 12/29/12 from
http://www.cdc.gov/physicalactivity/growingstronger/why/index.html

should be extremely encouraging for anyone who wants to incorporate strength training into his/her weekly routine.

## David Ratherdale, 65, with Type II Diabetes

Consider, first of all, David, who has made so much progress through strength training that he is able to control his diabetes with diet and exercise to the exclusion of insulin injections! Has he been pumping iron 24/7? Not at all. Let's take a look at his weekly routine.

For the past several years, David has been walking a two-mile course in his neighborhood, which takes him about 45 minutes. In addition to this walking, David has followed a simple regimen of strength training in his basement, performing three repetitions of squats and shoulder presses to work all of his major muscle groups.

Here is David's typical week:

- Sunday, Tuesday, Thursday, Saturday—45-minute walk
- Monday, Wednesday, Friday—Strength training

David has not only tamed his diabetes without insulin, he has lost 65 pounds and reports more positive emotions and higher energy levels. He says that the fear of the complications from diabetes, such as going blind or losing a foot, propels him out the door every other day for his walk or down into his basement to work out a bit. (Suitable exercises like the ones that David does will be detailed in chapter 3)

## Harold Moss, 67, Cancer Survivor

If the huge group of seniors that have diabetes can relate to David's story, then another giant group of seniors that have survived cancer can find common ground with Harold.

As a former tennis instructor, Harold was a bit more athletic in his younger years, and he has clung to tennis as the lifetime sport that it is. In addition to playing tennis and swimming, Harold does weight training in the fitness center of his apartment building, working on his biceps, triceps, quads, hamstrings and stomach muscles. (See chapter 3 for exercises like Harold's)

Here is a typical week in Harold's life:

- Sunday—an hour of tennis
- Monday—tennis plus strength training
- Tuesday—15-minute swim
- Wednesday—strength training
- Thursday—tennis
- Friday—swim and strength training
- Saturday—tennis

Harold says that after a period of physical "catastrophes", including high blood pressure, prostate cancer surgery and hip replacement, he felt like a shell of himself. He began strength training to speed his recovery from hip replacement surgery and continued lifting weights long after the procedure was done. He reports that he didn't lose weight for a long time despite this vigorous program, but that he recently trimmed 10 pounds off his frame.

### T. Boone Pickens, 83, Billionaire Investor

None of us think that we have much in common with T. Boone Pickens, the flamboyant billionaire that continues to preach against America's dependence on foreign oil. Yet, in his most recent book *The First Billion is the Hardest*, Pickens devotes a sizeable portion of his autobiography to the story of how he discovered strength training in his golden years.

Dragged down by low energy levels and constant stress, Pickens hired a personal trainer and began to work out in a gym five days a week, minimum. He felt so much better that he began a fitness program loaded with incentives in all of his corporate offices, building fitness centers into all of the office buildings that he controls.

Pickens now says that his strength training time is a sacred hour on his daily calendar that no executive can touch, and he shares much wisdom in his book regarding the increased need for strength training as we age, arguing against the normal decrease in physical activity that most seniors anticipate. Pickens believes that his strength training has enabled his mind to stay sharp into his 80s, and he wonders if he would even be alive today if he had not discovered the wonders of strength training.[21]

---

[21] *The First Billion is the Hardest: Reflections on a Life of Comebacks and America's Energy Future*, T. Boone Pickens, Crown Business, 2009.

## CHAPTER TWO

## A Program for Strength Training

In any new pursuit, it is important to control yourself as you seek to establish a new lifestyle. Perhaps you have read the previous pages and are ready to climb Mount Everest as proof of your deep motivation to improve your health. What you will find, if you literally or figuratively try to climb a mountain, is that you will be sore for days and possibly weeks due to overdoing your new exercise regime. That will mean many lost days of workouts and perhaps a total withdrawal from strength training.

It's far better to start slowly and build up strength. That is why most strength training programs are called progressive strength training routines.

On the other hand, you should not be so daunted by the routines described above or the mere thought of doing bicep curls that you never take action! The opposite of overdoing a new exercise routine is abstaining from it because of various fears or a lack of motivation. What you will find is that if you simply start with a few simple exercises that can actually be somewhat enjoyable, you can establish an unbreakable momentum that continues for a lifetime.

As you begin to see the positive results of your new strength training routine, you will become even more motivated to continue it.

Before getting into the specifics of strength training exercises, let us first establish just how much time you should put into this new routine. These guidelines have been established by the Centers for Disease Control and Prevention, and other sources.

## How Much Time Per Week Will Strength Training Require?

As you might guess, this varies from person to person. You probably should not aim for the bare minimum. That indicates a mind-set that is only partly committed to engaging in this new habit.

The good news is that benefits can result from as little as one day per week of strength training, especially when combined with other aerobic activities such as walking or swimming. However, the federal Department of Health and Human Services recommends that strength training be done at least two days per week, targeting all major muscle groups (legs, back, hips, chest, abdomen, shoulders, arms) and that your muscles are given at least one day's rest between strenuous exercises.

The length of strength training sessions should probably begin at about 20 minutes and then increase gradually to achieve a workout time of one hour, if possible.

If you are 65 or older and fairly fit with no limiting health conditions, here is the amount of time that you should spend exercising to begin to experience mental and physical benefits:

- Strength training for two days per week + two hours and 30 minutes of moderate-intensity aerobic activity such as walking
- Strength training for two days per week + one hour and 15 minutes of vigorous-intensity aerobic activity such as jogging
- Strength training for two days per week + two hours featuring a mix of moderate- and vigorous-intensity activity

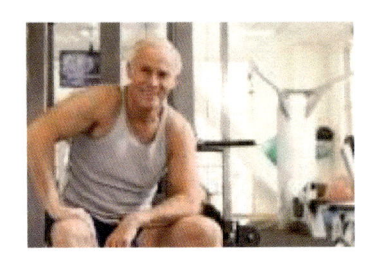

Seniors that have more time and energy can increase strength training to three days per week and do up to five hours of moderate-intensity aerobic activity. Do not think that you have to dedicate eight hours per week to become extremely fit. Start with an hour per week of strength training divided into two sessions and mix in two-plus hours of walking or just over an hour of jogging. This will be an excellent starting point for your first several months of exercise and can be tailored to fit most schedules.

**What Counts as Strength Training and Aerobic Activity?**

You don't even necessarily have to pump iron or jog a particular course to meet the exercise outline described above. Some common activities can qualify as strength training and aerobic activity.

Anything that gets you breathing hard and causes your heart to beat faster can be called aerobic activity. If you do any of the activities below for at least 10 minutes, you can chalk it up as part of your aerobic activity (moderate intensity) for the week:

- Pushing a lawn mower
- Participating in a dance class
- Biking to the store
- Walking at a moderately intense pace

As for strength training, it usually is best done with weights and specific movements that have been proven to give maximum results for targeted areas. These types of exercises are detailed in chapter 3. However, these activities can also count towards the time you spend on strength training:

- Heavy gardening
- Shoveling snow
- Some forms of yoga

**What You Will Need**

If you are going to work out at home, you will need a few pieces of equipment to perform all of the exercises listed in chapter 3. You should have:

- A sturdy chair with no arms
- Good athletic shoes
- Comfortable clothing that breathes as you perspire
- A pair of light dumbbells. Don't try to use homemade weights. The handles of a milk jug or other similar item could break and cause injury. Dumbbells are not very expensive. Buy a set of three different weights if possible so that you can progress in your training.
- Ankle weights, also not very expensive and can be used to increase resistance as you do various leg exercises.
- An exercise mat. This can provide extra cushioning for exercises that require you to lie on the ground.
- A storage container to keep your weights off the floor and keep people in your home from tripping over them and falling unnecessarily.

Obviously, you can join a nearby health club or YMCA and do your exercises in groups or under the supervision of a trainer. If you want to do your strength training in the comfort of your own home, then you will need the gear described above.

There are pros and cons to working out at home. You can do it at any time, but you lose the motivation that can be provided by others around you working out at the same time. You also might need professional guidance as you exercise. A trainer can really help you perfect the proper form for any movements that you do.

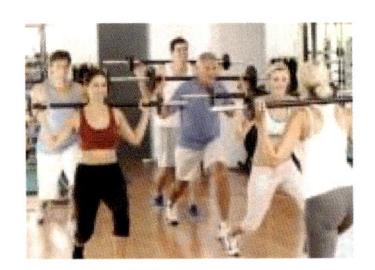

The exercises described in this e-book can be done at home or in a fitness center. The choice is yours.

**Helpful Steps before You Start Moving**

Many professionals who help others to begin and sustain strength training programs for their clients recommend a few preliminary steps before the actual lifting and stretching begin. Here are several actions that you might want to take before joining a gym or designating a room in your house as a workout area:

- Check with your doctor before embarking on a rigorous exercise routine, especially if you have a chronic disease, such as arthritis, diabetes, high blood pressure or a heart condition. Your doctor can advise the best type of strength training program for you in light of your physical limits.

- Take time to consider your reasons for engaging in strength training, the goals that you want to achieve and the potential obstacles that can keep you from meeting those goals
- Many exercise pros recommend visualization as an important pre-exercise routine. It has been proven that Olympic athletes, for instance, have achieved personal bests and superior results after engaging in visualization. For you as a senior about to dive into strength training, that could mean visualizing a taxing workout in your den that leaves you feeling energized and on the road to better health.
- Clearly spell out your goals, making them "SMART"=Specific, Measurable, Attainable, Relevant and Time-based. Perhaps your goal is one hour of strength training per week, focusing on your back. You can write out a goal with that specific aim. Or, perhaps it is getting back to doing all of your usual chores after recovering from surgery. The best goals feature a mix of short- and long-term objectives. Writing them down and posting them somewhere prominently can help you to sustain your motivation.
- Make a plan based on your goals to set up the ideal conditions for you to achieve them. That might involve buying some equipment or enrolling in a gym. It could mean taking a hard look at your weekly calendar or making a phone call to challenge a friend to be your workout buddy. Many studies have shown that exercise done in groups will be more easily sustained than solo programs

.

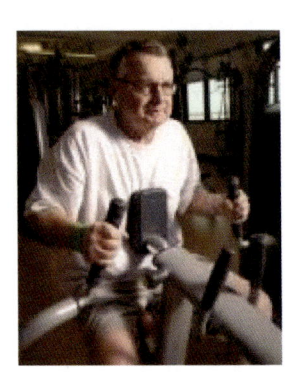

- Figure out a way to celebrate your achievements as goals are reached. When you attain three hours per week of exercise, buy yourself a new workout shirt or plan a scenic hike. Other personal rewards that can actually help to sustain your momentum in fitness can include buying new pieces of exercise equipment or clothing, massage time, dance class enrollment, new shoes or a vacation that will include different fitness challenges.
- Determine your present state of fitness to design a proper course of exercise. Numerous websites can help with this, including a checklist available here.
- Wait until you are relatively healthy to embark on a new strength training regime. That means that you should be free from cold, flu or fever; unusual pain or swelling; hernia, or any other unusual symptoms.
- In addition to ensuring that you have the right physical space in which to do strength training, you should also be sure that you are in a good place mentally to work out. That means finding spots in your schedule that will allow you to achieve maximum gains. For some, that is before work on weekday mornings; for others, that is during a favorite TV program each evening. Whatever slice of time you designate for strength training, be sure to give the muscles that you work the day off after moving them. You can do upper body work

one day and lower body work the next, for instance, or do all of your strength training on alternate days.
- It helps many people to write their strength training times into their schedules, either on paper or into a calendar on their electronic device. This helps to motivate them to keep their appointment with the dumbbells, just as they would for a visit to the doctor or dentist.
- Tweak your schedule as needed. Your weekly routine might vary, so you might need to change your workout times. You also should not be consumed by guilt if you miss a day or two due to illness or other commitments. Many healthy seniors do say, however, that they must treat their exercise time as a sacred time, or it will be swallowed up by other options.
- The saying "no pain, no gain" doesn't apply to strength training for seniors. You should feel strain as you perform many of the exercises in chapter 3, but if you feel consistent pain, you should not continue with a given movement. That is your body's way of telling you that you are overdoing it. Listen to your body and try a different exercise. Pain in your joints should especially be avoided while working out.

# CHAPTER THREE

## SUGGESTED EXERCISES AND APPROACH

Once you have been fully convinced of the many benefits of strength training for seniors and have composed reasonable goals and cleared some time out of your schedule to work out, it's time now to try a few exercises. This chapter will give you many options for your strength training workout. Pick the ones that meet the criteria that you establish, whether that be increased muscle mass, fun while doing the movement or focusing on a particular trouble spot, such as the lower back.

Any exercise period will proceed better if your muscles are warm. That is why most trainers prescribe a 5-10-minute walk to loosen up before engaging in strength training. This can be done outside, around the house or on a treadmill. Walking directs blood to your muscles and prepares your body for strenuous exercise. This warm-up will help to prevent injury because warm muscles will react better to the demands placed on them by weights. You can also warm up by biking a bit, hitting the rowing machine or stair stepper. At the conclusion of your workout time, you can do a similar cool-down by walking or biking.

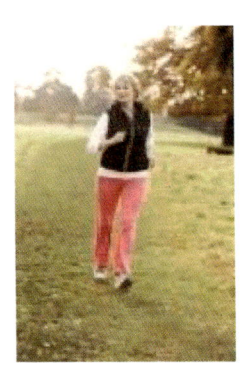

## Starter Exercises

Here is a sampling of starter exercises, to be done over the course of two weeks, for those who want to begin strength training and do not believe that they are fit enough to move directly into free weights, etc.:

- **Squats—great for strengthening hips, thighs and buttocks.**

To perform a set of squats, stand with your feet slightly more than shoulder-width apart in front of a sturdy chair with no arms, in position to sit in the chair. Extend your arms out, parallel to the ground and lean forward slightly at the hips.

Lower yourself in a slow and controlled motion with a count of four to a near –sitting position. Pause, then rise back up to a standing position with a count of two. Keep your back straight and your knees over your ankles, putting your weight on your heels, not the balls of your feet.

Repeat 10 times for one set, then rest for a minute or two and do a second set of 10.

If this squat is too difficult, place pillows in the chair or squat only four to six inches.

- **Wall Pushups—will strengthen the arms, shoulders and chest.**

Find a wall and stand a little more than one arm's length away.

Facing the wall, lean forward and place your palms flat against the wall at shoulder height, about shoulder-width apart.

As you count to four, bend your elbows and lower your upper body toward the wall in a slow and controlled motion, keeping your feet planted.

Pause, then push yourself back slowly away from the wall until your arms are straight, to a count of two. Don't lock your elbows.

Do one set of 10, pause for a minute or two, then do another set of 10. Do not arch your back during this exercise.

- **Toe Stands—strengthens calves and ankles and restores stability and balance.**

Near a counter or your sturdy chair, stand with your feet shoulder-width apart. Use the chair or counter for balance as you push your body up by standing on your toes, using your calves as you rise on the balls of your feet with a count of four.

Now, lower your heels back to the floor to a count of four.

Do one set of 10, pause for a minute or two, then do another set of 10. Don't lean on the counter or chair, and be sure to breathe regularly throughout this exercise.

- **Finger Marching—this three-movement exercise will strengthen your upper body and grip, and increase flexibility in your arms, back and shoulders.**

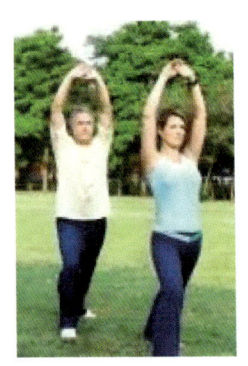

Stand or sit forward in your chair with feet on the floor, shoulder-width apart.

Imagine that there is a wall in front of you. Put your arms forward, palms facing outward, and walk your fingers up the imaginary wall until your arms are above your head.

Hold your arms above your head and wiggle you fingers for 10 seconds, then slowly walk them back down the imaginary wall.

Now, try to cross your arms behind your back, reaching your opposite elbow with each hand if possible. Hold for 10 seconds, then release your arms and wiggle your fingers as your hands come back out in front of your body.

This time, raise your arms until they are parallel to the ground, palms out, then interlock your hands and curl your shoulders forward to create a stretch in your upper back and wrist. Hold for 10 seconds.

Repeat these movements three times each with minimal pause between movements.

## Exercises for Those Ready to Use Weights

Perhaps you were already in fairly good shape before deciding to begin strength training. You might be the type of person who walks regularly, does tasks that require use of muscles, such as gardening or chopping wood, or you are already enrolled in a dance class at the local fitness center. If you fall into this category and do not consider yourself a beginner in fitness, then this next set of exercises will be at the proper intensity level for you.

If you embarked on this strength training quest and were not in shape, then you should be ready for these more demanding exercises after two weeks of doing the movements described above.

Here, then, is the next level of exercises as you continue to strength train regularly, to be bracketed by warm-up and cool-down of 5-10 minutes each:

- **Biceps curl—you will have no problem lifting items around the house after a few weeks of this exercise.**

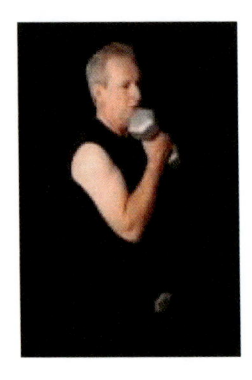

Either standing or sitting, with feet shoulder-width apart and arms at your sides, take a dumbbell in each hand, with your palms facing your thighs.

As you count to two, lift up the weights slowly and rotate your forearms so that your palms now face your shoulders. Keep your upper arms and elbows tucked to your side. Maintain straight wrists and keep the dumbbells parallel to the floor. Make sure that your arms, not your back, are doing the work.

Pause, then during a four-count, lower the dumbbells back down to your thighs, again rotating your forearms so that your palms face your thighs. This lowering is actually just as important as the raising of the dumbbells. Most people do not realize this when doing bicep curls. Proper form is essential to getting the maximum benefit of this exercise.

Do a set of 10, rest for a minute or two, then do a second set. Be careful of overdoing this exercise at first so that you can avoid extremely sore arms that can be quite painful for days. Don't let your enthusiasm get the best of you!

- **Step Ups—you will have better balance as a result of stronger legs, hips and buttocks after doing this exercise.**

You will need a set of stairs for this movement, preferably with a handrail.

Stand by a handrail at the bottom of a staircase with your feet flat and toes facing forward toward the stairwell. Now, put your right foot on the first step.

While holding the handrail, count to two as you straighten your right leg and lift up your left leg to the first step. Your right leg should be completely powering this movement.

Tap your left foot on the first step, then lower it back to the floor on a four-count.

Repeat 10 times with the right leg doing the lifting, then the left leg doing the heavy work. Rest for a minute or two and then do a set of 10 with each leg again.

Don't use your back leg at all while doing this movement, and do not let momentum do the work, either. Lean back on your heel as your leg is stressed. You will feel the burn much more than you could anticipate as you tax your leg muscles. This simple exercise will do wonders for your legs and help you to walk, climb stairs and do all sorts of other daily activities more easily.

- **Overhead Press—this will strengthen your arms, upper back and shoulders, and make reaching for objects in high places much easier.**

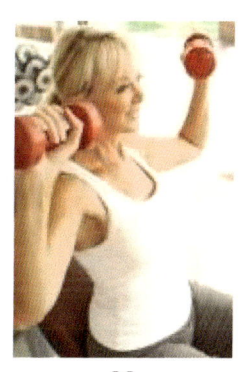

Stand or sit with feet shoulder-width apart. With a dumbbell in each hand and palms facing forward, raise them to shoulder height.

Then, as you count to two, raise the dumbbells over your head until your arms are fully extended. Do not lock your elbows.

Pause, then lower the dumbbells back to shoulder level as you count to four. Your elbows should be close to your sides. As with the biceps curl, this downward motion is equally important and vital to building muscle. Don't lower the weights too quickly.

Do a set of 10 raises, pause for a minute or two, then do a second set. Do not over-do this exercise, either, in the beginning. Keep your wrists straight and don't forget to breathe as you lift!

- **Hip Abduction—you can strengthen this very vulnerable area with this simple exercise.**

Standing behind your chair, put your hands on its back and keep your feet slightly apart with toes facing toward the chair. Don't lock your knees.

On a two-count, lift your right leg slowly to the side. Keep your left leg straight but don't lock the knee.

Pause, then count to four as you lower your right foot back to the ground.

Repeat 10 times with the right leg, then 10 times with the left leg. Rest for a minute or two before tackling a second set. Try your best not to lean as you do this movement. Add ankle weights to increase the difficulty if you'd like. You'll be surprised at how effective this exercise is!

### Additional Exercises

Once you have been doing the exercises in the second group described above for a month or so, you can now probably add other exercises to your routine. These additional exercises will work out different muscles all over your body. You will need a few more pieces of equipment to do some of them.

It is recommended that you build the number of exercises to the point where you can do about an hour of movement two or three times per week. It is also advised that you work several different muscle groups and not focus on biceps or thighs, for instance. A total body workout will give you the best chance to more easily do a wide variety of household tasks with greater ease.

Here, then, are several more exercises that you can fold into your routine. Don't forget that you can also work out 30-45 minutes every day if you alternate muscle groups, exercising your lower body on Mondays, Wednesdays and Fridays, for instance, while working your upper body on Tuesdays, Thursdays and Saturdays. Some people prefer this format to ensure that they are active each day; it is also convenient for people who have 30, rather than 60, minutes per day for exercise.

- **Knee Extension—this movement will strengthen your knees by building up the muscles around them. It is an excellent arthritis-fighter.** See the Knee Curl below for more help in building up this important area of your lower body.

If you have ankle weights, break them out for this exercise.

In your chair, sit with your feet grazing the ground. Sit on top of something if your feet are too flat on the ground.

Place your hands on your thighs and your feet about shoulder-width apart.

Point your toes forward and flex your foot. As you count to two, lift your right leg until the knee is straight.

Pause, then lower the leg slowly back to the ground during a four-count.

Repeat 10 times with the right leg, then 10 times with the left. Rest for a minute or two and then do a second set with each leg. This is a sort of leg press that you can do without going to the gym.

- **Knee Curl—this movement will strengthen the back of your upper leg (your hamstrings).** Be sure to do this exercise in conjunction with the knee extension above to bolster all the muscles in your upper leg.

Again, break out the ankle weights if you have them.

Stand behind your chair with your hands on its back, feet shoulder-width apart facing the chair.

As you flex your foot, bend your right leg back towards your buttocks, bringing the heel to touch if you can.

Pause, then lower the foot back to the ground during a four-count.

Repeat 10 times with the right leg, then 10 times with the left. Rest for a minute or two and continue on to a second set of 10 lifts with each leg. Keep the foot that is being raised in a flexed position at all times for maximum effect on the muscle.

- **Pelvic Tilt—this movement and others below will strengthen your core, which plays a much larger role in overall fitness than most people realize.**

Put your ankle weights away.

On a carpeted floor, thin mattress or exercise mat, lie flat on your back with knees bent, feet flat on the ground, arms at your side, palms down on the mat.

As you count to two, roll your pelvis upward so that the hips and lower back are off the ground. Your upper back and shoulders should still be on the ground during this movement.

Pause, then lower your pelvis back to the ground during a four-count.

Do this movement 10 times for a set, take a 1-2 minute break, then do a second set. Be sure to breathe normally throughout this exercise and keep your shoulders and upper back pinned to the ground.

- **Floor Back Extension—this is another great exercise for the core and provides relief for your lower back as abdominal muscles are strengthened.**

Lie on the floor or mat facedown, with two pillows under your hips.

Extend your arms straight out, parallel to the floor, as if you were about to dive into a pool.

On a two-count, lift your right arm and left leg off the floor, keeping them at the same level.

Pause, then lower both back to the floor during a four-count.

Do this 10 times for one set, then lift the left arm and right leg for another set of 10.

Rest for a minute or two and then do a second set of 10 reps for each leg. Keep your head, neck and back in a straight line throughout this exercise.

- **Abdominal Curl—this is another exercise that strengthens the core, which will help your posture and overall strength.**

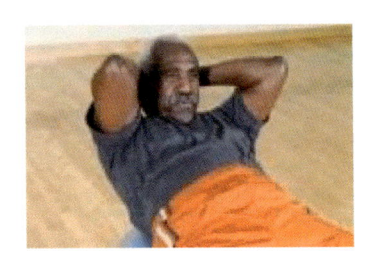

Lie on your back on a carpeted floor, firm mattress or exercise mat, feet flat and knees bent.

Place your hands behind your head with elbows pointing out, then slowly raise your shoulders and upper back off the ground while doing a two-count.

Pause, then lower your shoulders back down to the ground during a two-count.

Do one set of 10, rest for a minute or two, then do a second set of 10.

Breathe normally throughout this exercise and let your stomach muscles do the work, not your hands and arms pulling your head up. You also do not want to overdo this movement; sore abdominal muscles can make for several miserable days. This is an abbreviated sit-up.

- **Chest Press—using light dumbbells for this exercise will give your chest and shoulder muscles a good workout.**

Lie on your back on your mat, carpeted floor or firm mattress, with your knees bent and your feet flat.

Hold a dumbbell in each hand at chest level, shoulder-width apart, elbows bent and palms facing your knees.

Straighten your arms as you lift the dumbbells toward the ceiling, directly above your chest, while doing a two-count.

Pause, then lower the dumbbells back towards your chest during a four-count. This movement is just as important as the raising movement, so do not do it too quickly. Do this exercise with very controlled movements for maximum benefit. Do not allow your elbows to rest against the ground.

Repeat 10 times for one set, take a 1-2-minute break, then do a second set.

- **Lunge—this movement can greatly strengthen your upper leg and thighs.** Be careful with this one. It can work muscles that are not accustomed to being taxed, and it can be hard on the knees. Do this exercise only if you can perform it relatively free of pain.

Stand next to a counter or a chair with your feet shoulder-width apart. Hold on to the counter or chair with your right hand for balance.

Take a large step forward with your right foot and bend your right knee while you lower your hips toward the floor. Be sure that your right knee stays above your right ankle as you lower your body slowly.

Push against the floor with your right foot as you raise yourself up to your starting position.

Repeat 10 times with the right leg, then take a 1-2-minute break before doing a set with your left leg.

Remain as erect as possible as you do this exercise; don't lean forward or backward. The objective is for your front thigh to be parallel to the floor. Avoid sudden movements that can make your knee pop.

- **Upright Row—this movement will strengthen sometimes-little used muscles in the upper arms and upper back.**

Stand with your feet slightly spread and a dumbbell in each hand.

Palms should be facing your thighs with the dumbbells in front of your body at thigh level.

Raise the dumbbells in front of your body to shoulder height while doing a two-count, pulling them up as if you were rowing. Your elbows should be slightly higher than the dumbbells as you finish this movement.

Pause, then lower the dumbbells slowly during a four-count. This lowering is equally important to the exercise.

Do 10 reps for a set, take a 1-2-minute break and then do a second set.

Keep your back as straight as possible to ensure that the upper arms and upper back are doing the work in this movement.

- **Grip It—this exercise can help those who suffer from arthritis and have difficulty picking items up or maintaining a grip on them.** This movement can be done at any time, not just during your strength training session.

Take a racquetball, tennis ball or stress ball and squeeze it as hard as you can for 3-5 seconds.

Release the squeeze, pause, then repeat the squeeze 10 times for one set.

Do a second set, switch hands and do two sets of 10 with the other hand.

If you experience soreness or stiffness after this exercise, take at least one day off before doing it again.

All of the exercises above can be lengthened by performing a third set. It is not recommended that you do more than three sets. If you are able to do three sets easily, increase the amount of weight used when appropriate. Three sets will provide about five minutes of concentrated exercise, then you will be ready to move on to another exercise and not get bored.

## Stretching Exercises

As our bodies age, we get less limber. That is not news to anyone older than 30. Here are several exercises to stretch out various muscles in your body. They can be done as part of your cool down time or on a regular basis to keep yourself more limber.

- **Quadriceps Stretch—this movement will loosen up the muscles on the front of your thigh.** It can be done as part of a relaxation of the muscles after doing squats and other exercises that tax your upper leg.

Place your hands on the back of your chair or a countertop, with feet shoulder-width apart and knees slightly bent.

Bend your right leg back and grab your ankle with your right hand. This will require some flexibility on your part. If you are unable to do this movement, don't worry about it. Move on to other exercises. If, however, you can grasp your right ankle, pull your leg until your thigh is perpendicular to the ground. You should feel a stretching sensation at this point.

Hold this stretch for 30 seconds while maintaining normal breathing.

Release your right leg and do the same movement with your left leg. Relax throughout this exercise and don't lock your knees. Stand up straight for maximum benefit.

- **Hamstring/Calf Stretch—this movement will help you to bend over more easily.** These muscles are often the first to tighten as we age.

Sit in your chair with knees bent and feet flat on the floor.

Move your right leg out in front of you with your heel on the floor and your ankle relaxed.

Lean forward at the hips, bending towards your right toes while keeping your back straight and your knee unlocked.

Hold the stretch for 30 seconds while breathing normally.

Sit up straight again and flex the right ankle while your toes point upward. Lean again at the hips and hold the maximum stretch for 30 seconds again.

Release and repeat for two reps with the left leg.

Keep your back straight and your head lifted up as you lean forward. Don't overstretch and pull a muscle!

- **Chest and Arm Stretch—this exercise will enable your arms and chest to be more flexible for a variety of common movements.**

Stand with your arms at your sides and your feet shoulder-width apart.

Put your arms behind your back and clasp your hands together. Retract your shoulders if you can.

Hold the maximum stretch for 30 seconds.

Release the stretch and repeat.

Keep your back straight, breathe normally and look straight ahead. Concentrate on relaxing for maximum stretch.

- **Neck, Upper Back and Shoulder Stretch—these muscle areas often get the most tense. This stretch can help,** and you can do it at anytime during your day, not just during a strength training session.

Stand with your feet shoulder-width apart and knees bent slightly.

Clasp your hands in front of you.

Rotate your hands so that your palms are facing the ground, and raise your arms to chest height.

Press your palms away from your body. You should feel a stretching sensation in your neck, upper back and shoulders.

Hold the maximum stretch for 30 seconds.

Release and repeat with a straight back and normal breathing.

# CHAPTER FOUR

# MAKING PROGRESS

After following the counsel in chapter 2 and establishing a workable routine at least a couple of times per week by doing the exercises described in chapter 3, you might wonder what is next.

As you spend 1-3 months mastering the exercises in chapter 3 and discovering which ones you like the most and do the most good, you might even be up to one hour of strength training per session, and you could be repeating those sessions three times per week. Now, you are getting a little bored or wondering if you should make changes to your routine.

This is why the word "progressive" is often applied to strength training for seniors. In short, your strength training should be progressive.

You might make very slow progress, which is fine, but eventually you will want to increase the amount of weight that you use, the number of sets that you perform and perhaps even the variety of exercises that you build around to form your training sessions.

As you increase the intensity of your workout through greater weights or more numerous sets (up to three), you will be causing your muscles to grow stronger and stronger. The same goes for the stretching exercises in chapter 3. The more you stretch and the more often you stretch, the more limber you will become.

Progression in strength training is also important because it gives you a feeling of accomplishment. As you record your workouts in a journal, for example, you can note that you took a step up in weight used in month three. Progression can also help you to challenge yourself to reach greater heights in your strength training. You will be very proud of yourself for advancing from no weight used, for instance, to three pounds used in month nine. In any activity in life, making progress can give us an important sense of accomplishment and incentive to continue on the path that we have chosen.

Here are some simple tips for you as you seek to make progress in your strength training:

- Before you move onto heavier weights, be careful about your choice. If you are lifting an amount that is too heavy for you, injury can easily result. You could drop a dumbbell on your foot or tear a shoulder muscle when doing a movement with too much weight in your hand. Progress slowly and only lift when no significant pain is involved. Higher weight can also increase your blood pressure more than is needed.
- The optimal balance to achieve as you approach strength training is to make progress but also to prevent injury. Any progress that results in even minor injury is too rapid.

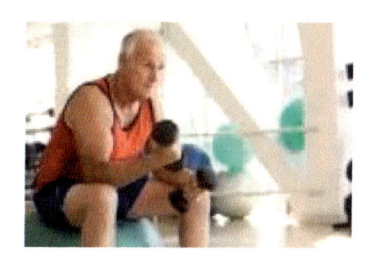

- A good test to decide if you can increase the amount of weight that you work with is this: can you do two sets of 10 reps in excellent form? If so, you can probably increase the amount of weight that you use, preferably in 1-lb. increments.
- Another good test to gauge the amount of weight that you should be using is this: if you need to rest between sets because the weight feels heavy, you are probably at the right amount of weight to be used. Do not plan on adding weight until you can do two sets almost consecutively.

- A good way to gradually work with increased weight is to do your first set at your normal weight, then do a second set with increased weight. Eventually, you will be able to do both sets with the increased weight.
- If you are unable to do at least eight repetitions in a set, then you have too much weight on your dumbbell.
- Ankle weights should be increased in ½-lb. amounts.

**Final Words**

We are all human beings with limited willpower and busy schedules. It might take you a few starts to incorporate regular strength training into your weekly routine. A lot of that will depend on how motivated you are and how completely you have bought into the points made in chapter 1 of this e-book.

If you truly believe that strength training can prolong your life, fight off dementia, make you happier and lengthen the amount of time that you can live independently, then you will probably find a way to do strength training regularly.

At other times in your life, you will have natural interruptions to your schedule. Don't get discouraged. It's often ironic how hard it can be to establish a regular exercise routine. It seems that the obstacles multiply when you make that first effort!

Persevere and pick up your routine after taking some time off for illness, vacation, family visiting your home over the holidays, etc. Depending on the length of your layoff, you might need to decrease the amount of weight that you use when you re-start your workouts.

No matter how many times you stop and re-start, you will be able to make up for lost ground. Thus, you should not get too discouraged or be too hard on yourself. If you have repeated interruptions that make regular workouts difficult to maintain, you might need to reassess your goals and plan accordingly. Some people have crowded schedules that vary from week to week; this can make regular exercise a true challenge.

Keep these three words in mind when you are tempted to give up altogether: "Healthy," "Strong," "Independent." Regular strength training can help you to achieve all three of these words over a lengthy period of time, making your golden years more enjoyable.

For more information on any of the points made in this e-book, consult the sources listed on the next page.

# SOURCES

http://www.cdc.gov/physicalactivity/growingstronger/index.html. This is a _great_ site with complete workout plans available and downloadable sheets that include motivational tips and space to record your workouts. You can watch videos of each exercise to ensure that you are using proper form; there are also many illustrations of the exercises described in this e-book.

http://www.eldergym.com/elderly-strength.html. Another great site with lots of info and exercises for your strength training program.

http://www.cfah.org/hbns/archives/getDocument.cfm?documentID=2091. One of many sites touting the benefits of strength training for seniors. Other documents are available at this site if you need more information or motivation.

http://health.usnews.com/health-news/news/articles/2012/04/23/strength-training-may-give-boost-to-seniors-brains. Another site with several articles about the wonders of strength training for seniors.

http://www.publicaffairs.ubc.ca/2010/12/13/strength-training-for-seniors-provides-sustained-cognitive-function-and-economic-benefits-vancouver-coastal-health-ubc-research/. A university website that contains results from studies that have been done on strength training for seniors. The various published papers make for interesting reading on the subject.

http://www.livestrong.com/article/105513-benefits-senior-strength-training/ Another good summary source that pulls from several different studies and articles, with typical Livestrong.com excellence.

Made in the USA
Lexington, KY
11 October 2013